Hue & Hustle
A GUIDE FOR ASPIRING MAKEUP ARTISTS
Of Color

Ordering Information:
Quantity sales. Special discounts are available on quantity purchases by corporations, associations, and others. For details, contact the publisher at the address above.

Printed in the United States of America

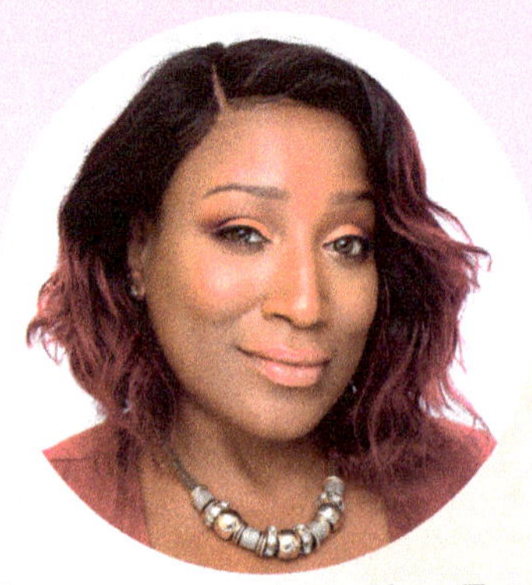

about

The Author

For over a decade, Trajean navigated the highs and lows of managing a successful makeup artistry business as an African American woman. Originating from the small town of Harrisburg, Pennsylvania, she faced numerous challenges due to the limited resources that more populous cities abundantly offer. In 1994, when she first ventured into the world of cosmetology, the path to becoming a makeup artist was obscure. Through diligent study and practice, drawing knowledge from industry veterans, Trajean honed her skills and built a reputation for crafting flawless, transformative looks. Trajean is excited to share all the lessons, now encapsulated in this book.

Today, Trajean is celebrated for her ability to treat each face as a unique canvas, enhancing individual beauty with every brushstroke. Her work spans a diverse global clientele, from everyday enhancements to bold fashion shoots. Beyond her artistry, she mentors aspiring makeup artists, sharing her journey and passion, inspiring others to explore the creative and expressive potential of makeup.

xoxo Trajean

Turn your Passion into Profit in the world of Makeup

table of Contents

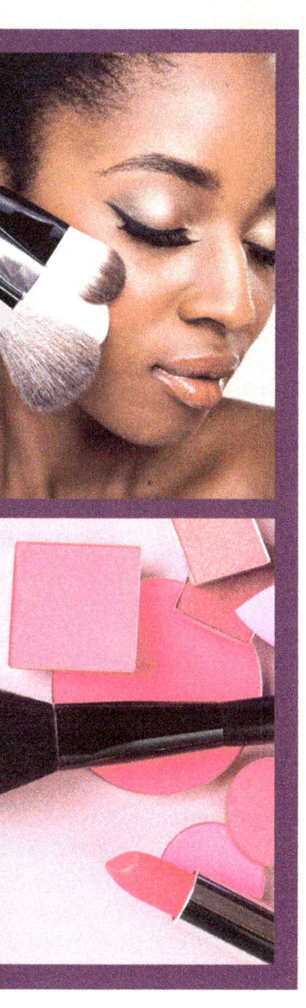

SETTING INTENTIONS

Before you turn the first page of "Hue & Hustle: A Guide For Aspiring Makeup Artists of Color" take a moment to set your intentions. Reflect on what drew you to the world of makeup artistry and what you hope to achieve through your journey in this creative field. Setting intentions can help you approach each chapter with a clear mind and a focused purpose, ensuring that you absorb the insights and wisdom that resonate most with your personal and professional goals. As you read, imagine the skills and knowledge you will gain as stepping stones towards fulfilling your dreams of becoming a skilled makeup artist, capable of transforming not just appearances but also enhancing self-esteem and confidence in others. Let this book be a guide and an inspiration as you embark on this exciting path, equipped with intention and a vision for your future.

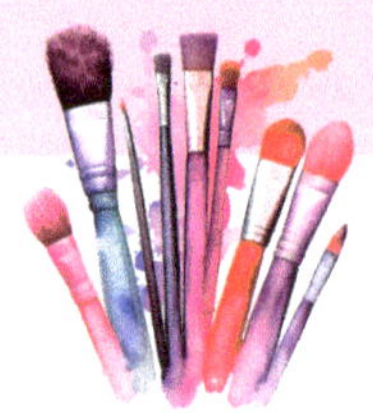

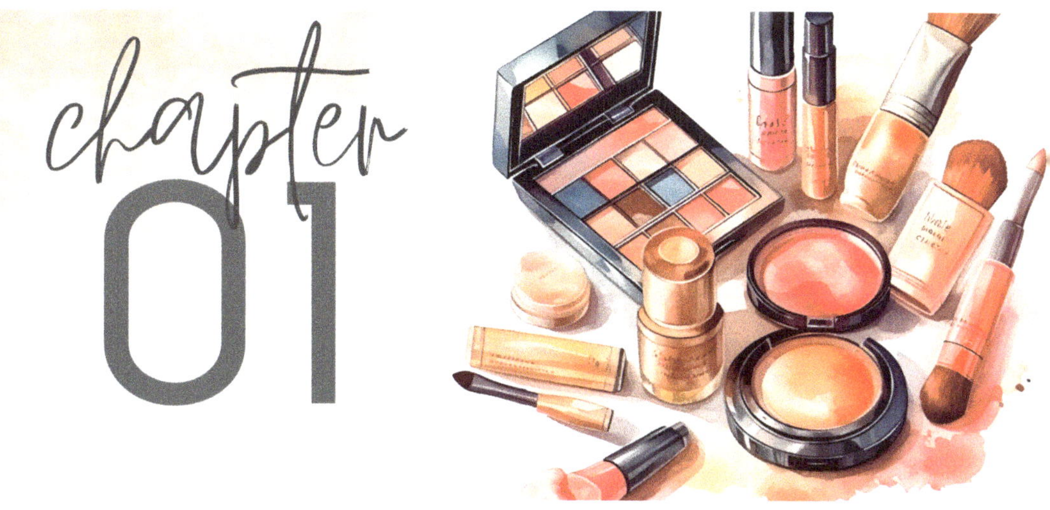

Welcome to the World of Makeup Artistry

Becoming a makeup artist is more than just applying makeup; it's about transforming faces, enhancing natural beauty, and expressing creativity through the art of cosmetics. As an African-American makeup artist, you bring a unique perspective and set of skills that are invaluable to the beauty industry. This chapter will introduce you to the journey ahead, highlighting the importance of passion, perseverance, and a clear understanding of your goals.

The Power of Makeup

Makeup has the power to boost confidence, express individuality, and transform appearances. It can turn a simple look into a statement, a mood, or a work of art. As a makeup artist, you'll have the opportunity to work with diverse clients, helping them achieve their desired look for various occasions, from everyday wear to special events.

Embracing Your Unique Perspective

Your identity as an African-American makeup artist is a powerful asset. The beauty industry is becoming increasingly inclusive, recognizing the need for diverse representation and expertise. Your background and experiences provide you with a unique lens through which you view and apply makeup. Embrace this perspective and let it shine through in your work, setting you apart in a crowded field

The Importance of Passion

Passion is the driving force behind every successful makeup artist. It fuels your creativity, motivates you to improve your skills, and keeps you resilient in the face of challenges. Your love for makeup artistry will be evident in your work and will attract clients who appreciate your dedication and talent.

Setting Clear Goals

Before diving into the technical aspects and business strategies of makeup artistry, it's crucial to set clear, achievable goals.

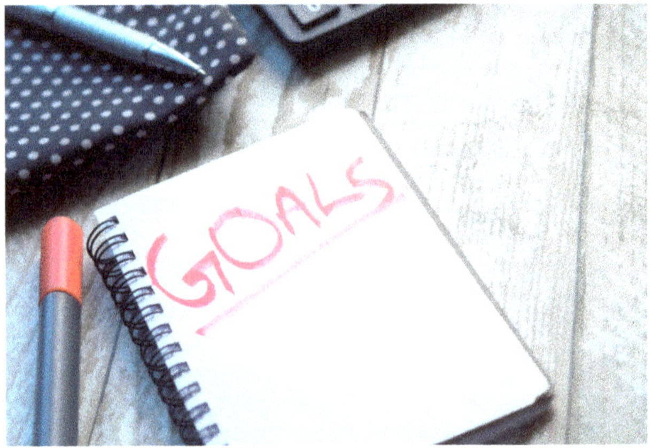

CLEAR GOALS

These goals will guide your journey and help you measure your progress. Consider the following questions as you define your goals:

What Kind of makeup Artist do you want to be?

Do you want to specialize in bridal makeup, fashion, editorial, special effects, or everyday beauty?

Who is your target audience?

Are you aiming to serve a particular demographic or offer your services to a broad range of clients?

What are your career aspirations?

Do you want to work as a freelance artist, join a beauty brand, or open your own studio?

Remember, every great journey begins with a single step. Your passion and dedication are your greatest assets. Stay focused, keep learning, and don't be afraid to take risks. The world of makeup artistry is waiting for your unique touch.

Understanding the Industry Landscape

The beauty industry is vast and constantly evolving. Staying informed about current trends, new products, and industry developments is essential. Here are a few aspects of the industry to keep in mind:

- **Trends**: Makeup trends change frequently. Keep up with the latest looks by following fashion shows, beauty influencers, and industry publications.

- **Products:** New products and innovations are regularly introduced. Stay updated on the latest releases and test products to understand their benefits and applications.

- **Techniques:** Continuous learning is key. Attend workshops, take online courses, and practice new techniques to enhance your skills.

- **Diversity and Inclusion:** The push for diversity and inclusion in the beauty industry is more prominent than ever. As an African-American makeup artist, you can contribute to this movement by promoting and celebrating diversity in your work.

Building a Strong Foundation

This book will provide you with the tools and knowledge to build a strong foundation for your career. From developing essential skills and creating a standout portfolio to understanding the business side of makeup artistry, each chapter is designed to guide you step-by-step.

chapter 02

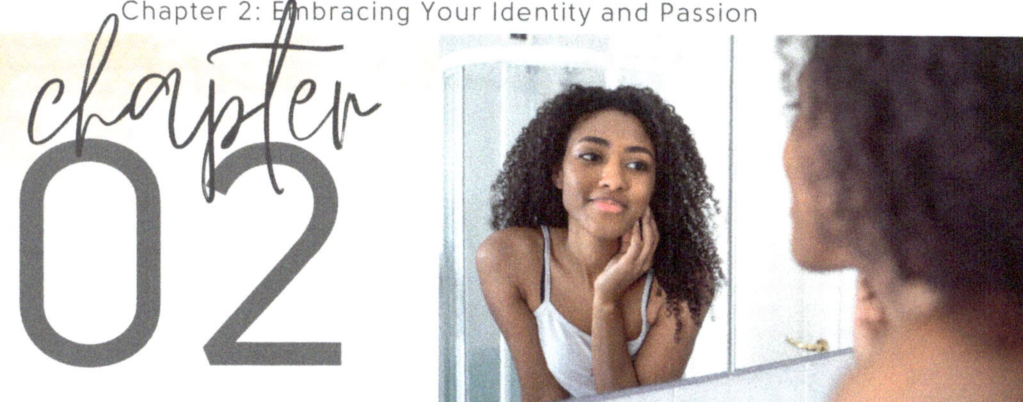

Discovering Your Unique Identity

As an African-American makeup artist, your identity is not just a part of who you are; it's a significant aspect of your brand and artistic expression. The beauty industry is gradually recognizing the importance of diversity and inclusion, but there is still much work to be done. Your unique perspective and experiences can contribute to this positive change and help fill the representation gap.

Celebrating Your Culture

Your culture and background provide a rich tapestry of inspiration. From traditional styles and colors to contemporary expressions of beauty within the African-American community, you have a vast reservoir of ideas to draw from. Incorporate elements of your heritage into your work to create looks that resonate with a wide audience while staying true to your roots.

Breaking Stereotypes

Unfortunately, the beauty industry has long been plagued by stereotypes and limited representations of beauty. As an African-American makeup artist, you have the power to challenge and break these stereotypes. Showcase the versatility and beauty of diverse skin tones and facial features through your work. This not only empowers your clients but also educates others and promotes inclusivity.

The Role of Passion in Your Journey

Passion is the foundation of any successful career, and makeup artistry is no exception. Your love for makeup and beauty will drive you to continually improve your skills, stay updated with industry trends, and provide exceptional service to your clients.

Finding Your Passion

To truly excel in makeup artistry, you need to understand what aspects of the field ignite your passion. Here are a few questions to help you identify your passions within makeup artistry:

- What excites you most about applying makeup?

- Do you enjoy creating bold, dramatic looks or prefer natural, everyday makeup?

- Are you drawn to specific types of makeup, such as bridal, editorial, or special effects?

- What inspires you when you think about makeup and beauty?

By answering these questions, you can pinpoint the areas where your passion lies and focus your efforts on honing those skills.

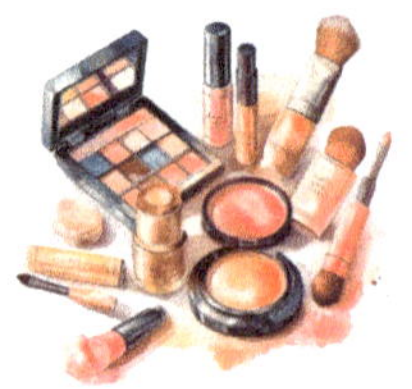

Fueling Your Passion

Passion needs to be nurtured and sustained. Here are some ways to keep your passion for makeup artistry alive:

- **Stay Curious**: Continuously explore new techniques, products, and trends. Never stop learning and experimenting.

- **Seek Inspiration**: Follow other makeup artists, attend beauty events, and immerse yourself in different forms of art and culture.

- **Practice Regularly**: The more you practice, the better you become. Make time for regular practice sessions to refine your skills.

- **Engage with the Community**: Join online forums, social media groups, and professional organizations where you can connect with like-minded individuals.

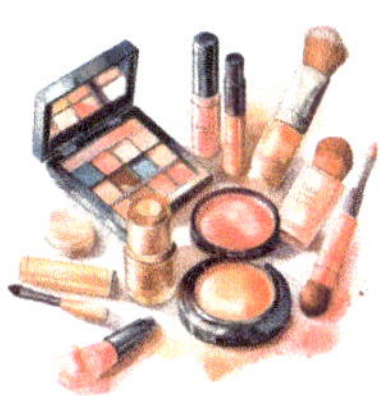

Building Confidence

Confidence is key to success in any field, and makeup artistry is no different. As you embark on your journey, it's important to build and maintain confidence in your abilities.

Overcoming Self-Doubt

Self-doubt can be a significant barrier, especially when starting out. Here are some strategies to overcome it:

- **Acknowledge Your Progress**: Celebrate your achievements, no matter how small. Recognize your growth and improvement over time.

- **Seek Feedback**: Constructive feedback from peers and mentors can help you identify areas for improvement and build confidence in your strengths.

- **Practice Self-Care**: Taking care of your mental and physical well-being is crucial. Ensure you have a healthy work-life balance and engage in activities that make you happy.

- **Surround Yourself with Support**: Build a network of supportive friends, family, and colleagues who believe in your talent and encourage you to pursue your dreams.

"when you support a small business, you support a dream."- Anonymus

Using Your Identity and Passion to Stand Out

In a competitive industry, your identity and passion are your greatest assets. Here are some ways to leverage them:

- **Develop a Signature Style**: Create a unique style that reflects your background and interests. This will help you stand out and attract clients who resonate with your work.

- **Tell Your Story**: Share your journey and the inspiration behind your work on social media, your website, and other platforms. Personal stories create connections and make you more relatable.

- **Educate and Advocate**: Use your platform to promote diversity and inclusivity in the beauty industry. Educate your audience about the importance of representation and advocate for positive change.

Embracing your identity and passion as an African-American makeup artist is essential for your success and fulfillment in this field. Your unique perspective and love for makeup are powerful tools that can help you stand out, inspire others, and drive positive change in the industry. As you continue your journey, remember to stay true to yourself, celebrate your culture, and let your passion guide you.

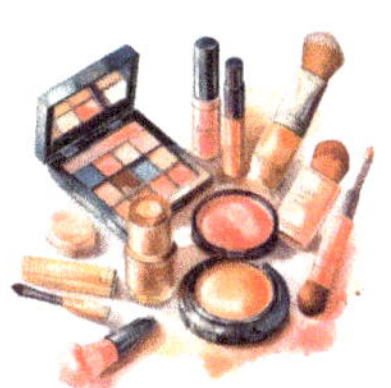

MORNING MOTIVATION

A morning motivation routine sets a positive tone for the day, energizing your focus and aligning your actions with your business goals, ensuring every step you take is intentional and productive. Here is a great one to try

Set the Tone for Your Day:

- Start with Gratitude: Begin each morning by listing three things you are grateful for. This can shift your mindset to one of positivity and abundance, making it easier to tackle the day's challenges.
- Morning Meditation: Spend 5-10 minutes in meditation, focusing on your breath or a specific intention for the day. This helps center your thoughts and reduces stress.
- Visualize Success: Take a few minutes to visualize your goals as already achieved. Imagine the feelings of success and the steps you took to get there. This visualization can enhance your motivation and clarity for the day ahead.
- Physical Activity: Engage in at least 15 minutes of physical activity, whether it's stretching, yoga, or a quick workout. This increases energy levels and improves focus.
- Nourishing Breakfast: Fuel your body with a healthy breakfast that energizes you without weighing you down. Include proteins, healthy fats, and fibers to keep you satisfied and alert.
- Review Your Goals: Take a moment to review your short-term and long-term goals. Adjust your daily to-do list to ensure it aligns with these goals, helping you stay on track to achieving your dreams.

Incorporating these steps into your morning routine can energize and prepare you to pursue your dreams with intention and vigor each day.

INSPIRING AFRICAN-AMERICAN MAKEUP ARTISTS

Pat McGrath

When I think about Black excellence in the beauty industry, Pat McGrath is the name that immediately comes to mind. As a 40-year-old Black woman who grew up in a low-income household, seeing someone who looks like me reach the pinnacle of success in the beauty world is nothing short of inspiring.

Pat McGrath's journey is a testament to the power of passion, creativity, and relentless determination. Born in Northampton, England, to a single mother who nurtured her artistic inclinations, Pat didn't have an easy path. Her mother, Jean McGrath, was a dressmaker who had a keen eye for fashion and beauty. She instilled in Pat a love for bold colors and unique styles, despite the financial challenges they faced. This foundation of creativity and resilience is something I deeply resonate with.

Growing up, makeup wasn't just about looking good; it was about expression and confidence. For Pat, it was a similar story. She didn't have access to the luxuries many others took for granted, but she made do with what she had, often using her mother's makeup to experiment with different looks. This ingenuity is something many of us from low-income backgrounds understand well – we learn to make the most out of very little.

INSPIRING AFRICAN-AMERICAN MAKEUP ARTISTS

Pat McGrath

Pat's big break came when she moved to London and began working with top photographers and designers. Her groundbreaking work in the 1990s, especially her collaboration with Edward Enninful for i-D magazine, set her apart as a visionary. She didn't just follow trends; she created them. Her work was a celebration of diversity and inclusivity long before it became a buzzword in the industry.

In 2015, Pat launched her own line, Pat McGrath Labs, which has since become a global phenomenon. For someone like me, who often felt underrepresented in mainstream beauty, Pat's products were a revelation. They cater to all skin tones, celebrating the richness and diversity of Black beauty. Her success story shows that it's possible to break barriers and redefine standards, no matter where you come from.

What I admire most about Pat McGrath is her commitment to authenticity. She has never shied away from her roots, always crediting her mother's influence and her humble beginnings. She embodies the belief that greatness can emerge from any circumstance, a powerful reminder for those of us who have had to fight for every opportunity.

Pat McGrath's legacy is more than just her incredible products; it's about changing the narrative for Black women in beauty. She's a beacon of hope and a symbol of what we can achieve with passion and perseverance. Her story motivates me to chase my dreams unapologetically, knowing that the sky is truly the limit.

chapter 03

Navigating the Beauty Landscape as an African-American Makeup Artist

The journey to becoming a successful African-American makeup artist is filled with both rewards and challenges. This chapter will delve into common obstacles you may face in the beauty industry and provide strategies to overcome them, ensuring your path is both progressive and fulfilling.

Common Challenges

Limited Representation

One of the most persistent challenges is the lack of representation. African-American artists and clients are often underrepresented in beauty campaigns, product ranges, and industry leadership.

Strategies to Overcome

- **Showcase Diversity in Your Portfolio:** Actively include a diverse range of skin tones and beauty styles in your work to demonstrate versatility and advocacy for broader representation.

- **Support and Collaborate**: Engage with other African-American professionals in the industry to build a supportive community that champions diversity.

Access to Opportunities

Access to high-profile gigs, networking events, and career-building opportunities can sometimes be more limited for African-American makeup artists.

Strategies to Overcome

- **Create Your Own Opportunities:** Launch independent projects or collaborate with other creatives to gain visibility and build your portfolio.

- **Utilize Digital Platforms**: Leverage social media and online marketing to reach a wider audience and showcase your skills.

- **Educate and Advocate**: Use your platform to promote diversity and inclusivity in the beauty industry. Educate your audience about the importance of representation and advocate for positive change.

Facing Bias

Bias, whether unconscious or overt, can affect hiring decisions, client interactions, and overall career progression.

Strategies to Overcome

- **Educate Clients and Peers**: Use your platform to inform about the beauty and versatility of all skin tones.

- **Seek Fair Treatment**: Don't hesitate to advocate for yourself and seek environments that value diversity and inclusion.

Building Resilience

Overcoming challenges in any career requires resilience—the ability to recover from setbacks and continue pushing forward.

Developing a Thick Skin

Criticism and rejection can be part of the job, but it's important to distinguish between constructive feedback and negativity.

Sustaining Motivation

- **Focus on Learning**: View each critique as an opportunity to learn and grow, not as a personal attack.

- **Stay Positive**: Keep a positive mindset and remember your successes and strengths.

Tips for Resilience

Maintaining motivation can be tough, especially when faced with industry barriers.

Tips for Staying Motivation

- **Set Small, Achievable Goals**: This helps create a sense of progress and accomplishment.

- **Celebrate Milestones**: Recognize and celebrate your successes to boost morale.

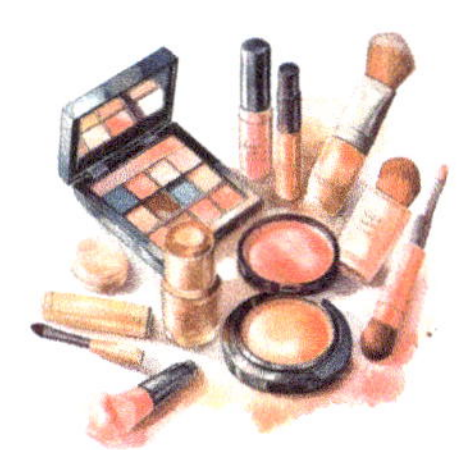

Advocating for Change

As an African-American makeup artist, you have the power to effect change in the beauty industry. Your success and visibility can inspire others and contribute to a more inclusive and equitable field.

Promoting Diversity

Emphasize the importance of diversity in your work and interactions. Collaborate with brands and platforms that support inclusivity.

Advocacy Actions

- **Speak at Events**: Share your experiences and insights on panels and at conferences.

- **Participate in Workshops**: Teach and learn in settings that promote diverse beauty standards.

Leveraging Influence

As you build your reputation, use your influence to advocate for broader changes in the industry, such as more inclusive product ranges and diverse advertising campaigns.

Leveraging Strategies

- **Partner with Brands**: Work with brands that are committed to diversity.

- **Use Social Media**: Regularly post about issues related to diversity and inclusion, highlighting the need for change.

Conclusion

Overcoming challenges as an African-American makeup artist is not only about advancing your own career but also about paving the way for future generations. By tackling obstacles with determination, advocating for inclusivity, and using your platform for change, you contribute to a more diverse and welcoming beauty industry.

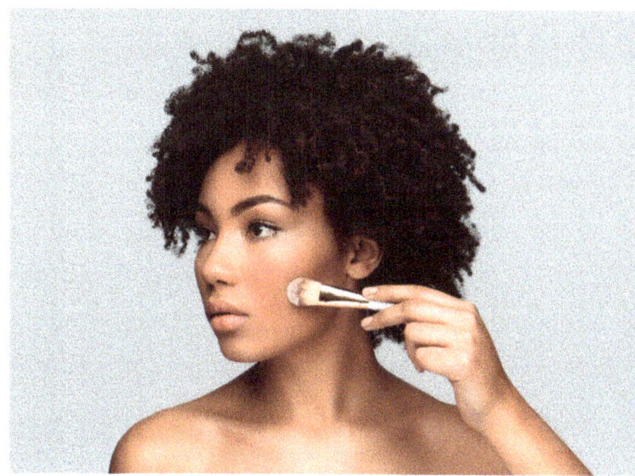

Building a Strong Foundation

As you forge your path in the makeup industry, developing a robust set of skills and acquiring the right education are crucial. This chapter explores the essential skills every makeup artist should master and the educational pathways that can enhance your expertise and credibility.

Mastering Makeup Techniques

To excel as a makeup artist, certain fundamental skills are indispensable:

Core Skills

- **Color Theory**: Understanding color theory is essential for creating harmonious makeup looks. Knowing how colors interact and contrast can help you enhance natural features and correct imperfections.
- **Skin Care Knowledge**: A good makeup application starts with skin care. Familiarity with different skin types and conditions allows you to prepare the skin properly before makeup and recommend suitable products.
- **Application Techniques**: From blending foundations to creating sharp eyeliner looks, your hand skills need to be precise and adaptable to different styles and occasions.
- **Understanding of Lighting**: Lighting can significantly affect how makeup appears. Knowledge of lighting helps you adjust makeup for various environments, whether it's a photoshoot or an indoor event.

Advanced Techniques

As you grow in your career, consider learning advanced techniques that can set you apart:

- **Special Effects Makeup**: For work in film, theater, or themed events, special effects makeup skills can be incredibly valuable.

- **Airbrushing**: Airbrush makeup application is popular for bridal and TV work because of its durability and smooth finish.

- **Historical Makeup Styles**: Knowledge of different historical makeup styles can be useful for themed photoshoots and period productions.

Educational Pathways

Formal Education

While not always mandatory, formal education in makeup artistry can give you a competitive edge:

- **Makeup Schools**: Enrolling in a reputable makeup academy offers structured learning and hands-on experience. It can also provide valuable certifications.

- **Workshops and Seminars**: Regularly attending workshops and seminars keeps you updated with the latest techniques and products.

- **Online Courses**: Many renowned makeup artists offer online courses, which are a flexible way to learn from industry leaders.

Continous Learning and Improvement

Staying Current

The beauty industry evolves rapidly, and staying informed about the latest trends and techniques is crucial:

- **Industry Publications**: Subscribe to beauty and fashion magazines and follow relevant blogs and YouTube channels.

- **Trade Shows and Expos**: Attending beauty trade shows and expos can provide insights into emerging trends and new products.

- **Networking**: Engaging with other professionals can lead to mentorship opportunities and insider knowledge on industry advancements.

Building a Professional Portfolio

Showcase Your Skills

Your portfolio is a critical tool in attracting clients and demonstrating your capabilities:

- **Quality Over Quantity**: Include only your best work that showcases a variety of styles and techniques.

- **Professional Photos**: Invest in professional photography to make sure your work is presented in the best light.

- **Digital Presence**: In today's digital age, having an online portfolio is essential. Use platforms like Instagram or a personal website to display your work.

Certification and Licensing

The Importance of Credentials

Depending on where you plan to work, certification or licensing might be required:

- **State Licensing:** Some states in the U.S. require makeup artists to have a cosmetology or esthetician license, especially if you work with skin treatments.

- **Certifications**: Even if not required, certifications from recognized institutions can enhance your resume and instill trust in potential clients.

Conclusion

Building a successful career in makeup artistry requires a mix of technical skills, continuous education, and professional development. By mastering essential techniques, staying updated on industry trends, and showcasing your work effectively, you position yourself as a knowledgeable and versatile makeup artist. Always remember, the beauty of your career is largely dependent on the depth of your skills and the clarity of your educational pursuits.

Up next, learn about "Building Your Portfolio," where we'll delve into the best practices for creating a compelling and professional portfolio that attracts clients and showcases your unique artistic vision.

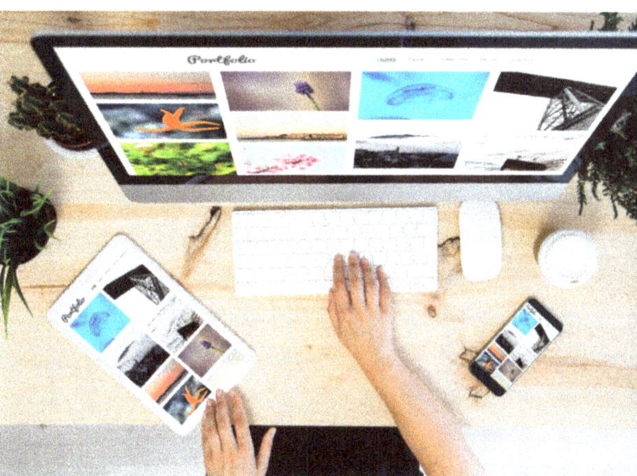

Crafting Your Professional Showcase

Your portfolio is more than a collection of your work; it's a reflection of your artistry, versatility, and professionalism. This chapter provides insights into creating a compelling portfolio that not only showcases your skills but also appeals to a broad range of clients.

Understanding the Importance of a Portfolio

A well-crafted portfolio is crucial for making a good first impression. It demonstrates your expertise in various makeup styles and techniques, helping potential clients and employers see your potential.

Goals of a Professional Portfolio

- **Demonstrate Versatility**: Show a range of styles from natural to avant-garde to appeal to diverse clients.

- **Highlight Skill Level**: Showcase your best work that speaks to your expertise and attention to detail.

- **Reflect Personal Brand**: Ensure your portfolio aligns with your branding, emphasizing your unique artistic voice.

Selecting Your Best Work

Choosing which pieces to include can be challenging. Here are some guidelines to help you curate your portfolio effectively:

- **Quality Over Quantity**: It's better to have fewer high-quality images than many mediocre ones.

- **Diversity**: Include work that shows a range of techniques, styles, and client demographics.

- **Recent Works**: Make sure your portfolio is up-to-date with current trends and your latest skills.

Professional Presentation

How you present your portfolio can be just as important as the content itself.

Physical Portfolio

- **High-Quality Prints**: Use professional-grade prints and a well-organized, stylish portfolio case.

- **Consistent Layout**: Arrange your work in a logical order that tells a story or groups similar styles together.

Digital Portfolio

- **Website**: Create a professional website with an easy-to-navigate gallery of your work.

- **Social Media**: Utilize platforms like Instagram to create a digital portfolio that can reach a global audience.

- **Online Portfolio Platforms**: Consider using sites like Behance or LinkedIn to showcase your work professionally.

Enhancing Your Portfolio with Collaborations

Working with other professionals can enhance the quality and diversity of your portfolio.

Collaboration Benefits

- **Professional Photography**: Work with photographers to ensure your makeup looks are captured with high quality.

- **Diverse Models**: Collaborate with models of various ages, skin tones, and features to showcase your versatility.

- **Stylists and Designers**: Teaming up with clothing stylists or fashion designers can lead to more polished and cohesive looks.

Updating and Reviewing

Your portfolio is a dynamic tool that should evolve as you grow in your career.

Regular Updates

- **Add New Work**: Continuously update your portfolio with new work to keep it fresh and relevant.

- **Remove Older Pieces**: As you improve, replace older works with newer ones that better showcase your skills.

- **Seek Feedback**: Regularly seek feedback from peers, mentors, or clients to understand how your portfolio can be improved.

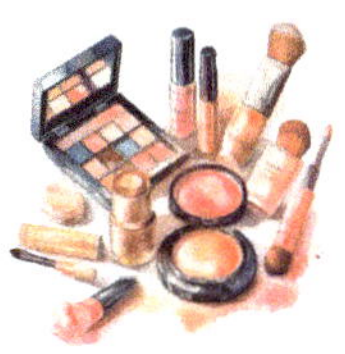

Leveraging Your Portfolio for Opportunities

A great portfolio opens doors to new opportunities.

Collaboration Benefits

- Job Applications: Tailor your portfolio for specific job applications to show relevance and customization.

- Client Meetings: Bring your portfolio to client meetings to illustrate your capabilities and discuss potential looks.

- Marketing: Use your portfolio in marketing materials to attract new business and partnerships.

Conclusion

Your portfolio is one of your most valuable marketing tools as a makeup artist. It serves as a tangible representation of your artistry and professionalism. By carefully curating and regularly updating your work, you can attract the right clients and opportunities that will help you build a successful career. Always remember, the strength of your portfolio can significantly influence your professional trajectory.

Next, delve into "Networking and Building Relationships," where you'll learn strategies to expand your professional network and foster relationships that can lead to career advancement and collaborative opportunities.

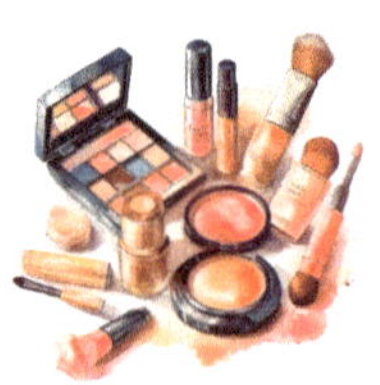

 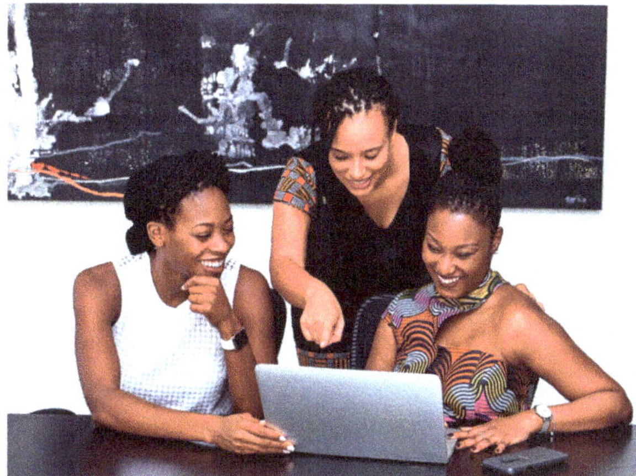

The Power of Professional Connections

In the makeup industry, who you know can be as important as what you know. This chapter focuses on how to effectively network and build relationships that can lead to career opportunities, collaborations, and growth.

Understanding Networking

Networking involves creating and maintaining professional relationships that are mutually beneficial. It's not just about meeting people; it's about connecting on a level that could lead to future opportunities, advice, and support.

Benefits of Networking:

- **Opportunity Access:** Networking can lead to job offers, freelance gigs, and collaborative projects that might not be advertised publicly.

- **Learning and Growth**: Relationships with peers and mentors provide invaluable learning opportunities and feedback.

- **Visibility**: Regular interaction with industry professionals keeps you top of mind for opportunities and recommendations.

Effective Networking Strategies

Attend Industry Events

Makeup shows, beauty expos, and workshops are perfect venues for meeting people in your field. Make an effort to:

- **Prepare**: Know who will be attending and prioritize whom you want to meet.

- **Engage**: Start conversations, exchange contact information, and follow up after the event.

Utilize Social Media

Platforms like LinkedIn, Instagram, and Facebook are excellent tools for networking.

- **Active Engagement**: Regularly post updates, comment on others' posts, and join relevant groups.

- **Professional Profile**: Ensure your social media profiles are professional and reflect your work and personality.

Join Professional Associations

Being part of professional beauty associations can provide networking opportunities, resources, and credibility.

- **Membership Benefits**: Attend conferences, participate in workshops, and access member-only resources.

- **Volunteer**: Offer to help with events and committees to increase visibility and connections.

Building Meaningful Relationships

Quality Over Quantity

It's better to have a few meaningful relationships than many superficial ones. Focus on connections that offer mutual growth and support.

Follow-Up and Consistency

- **Regular Contact**: Keep in touch with your contacts through emails, social media, or meetings.

- **Add Value**: Always think about how you can help others. This could be through referrals, advice, or support.

Mentorship

Finding a mentor in the makeup industry can accelerate your career and provide guidance through its complexities.

Finding a Mentor:

- **Identify Prospective Mentors**: Look for professionals whose careers inspire you.

- **Formal vs. Informal Mentorship**: Some relationships naturally evolve into mentorships, while others might be formalized through programs.

Being a Good Mentee:

- **Be Engaged**: Show interest and initiative in learning.

- **Respect Time:** Understand your mentor's time is valuable. Be punctual and prepared for meetings.

Collaborations

Working on projects with other professionals can help you learn, grow, and expand your portfolio.

Tips for Successful Collaborations:

- **Clear Communication**: Discuss goals, responsibilities, and expectations upfront.

- **Professionalism**: Treat every collaboration as a professional commitment.

- **Show Appreciation**: Always thank your collaborators and acknowledge their contributions.

Networking Challenges

Overcoming Introversion

- **Preparation**: Prepare talking points and questions in advance to ease anxiety.

- **Small Settings**: Start with smaller events or one-on-one meetings if large gatherings are intimidating.

Navigating Competitive Environments

- **Focus on Collaboration**: Emphasize mutual benefits and shared goals in your interactions.

- **Stay Positive**: Maintain a positive, professional attitude, even in competitive settings.

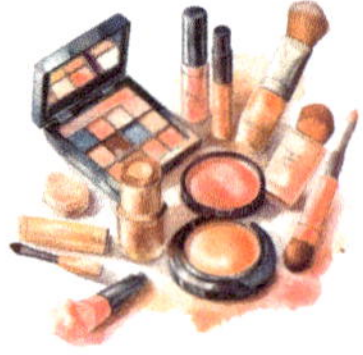

Conclusion

Networking and building relationships are foundational elements of a successful career in makeup artistry. By actively engaging with your peers, seeking mentorship, and collaborating on projects, you can create a supportive network that propels you toward your professional goals. Remember, every interaction is an opportunity to learn, grow, and potentially open doors to new possibilities.

Next, we explore "Marketing and Branding Yourself," where you'll learn to effectively promote your unique skills and style to attract and retain clients in a competitive market.

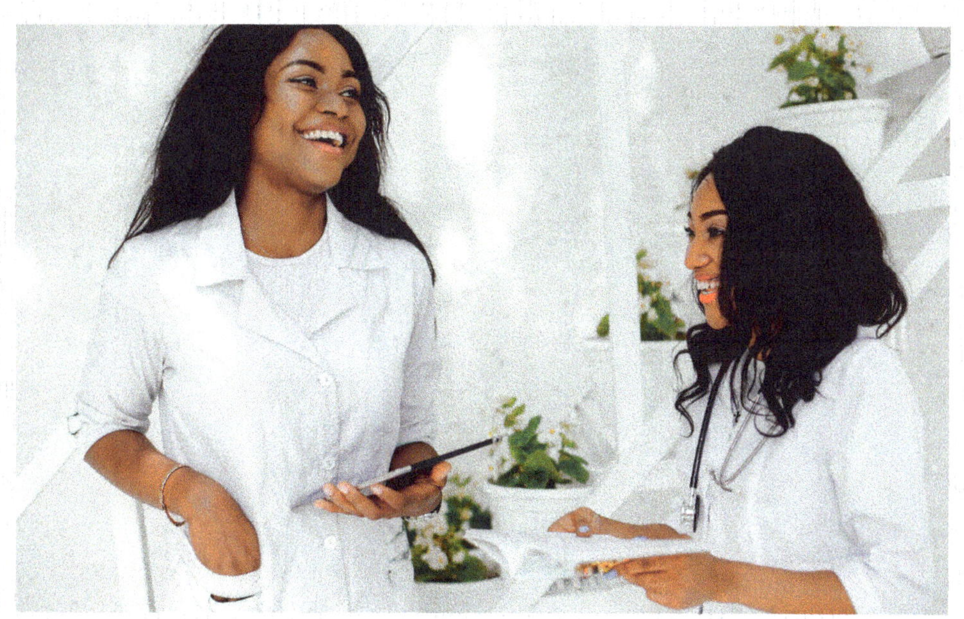

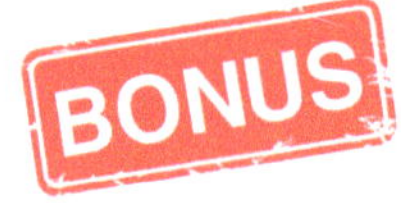

VISION BOARDS

Starting a vision board for your business is a powerful tool to bring clarity and focus to your entrepreneurial journey. By visually representing your goals and aspirations, you can keep your ambitions in sight and stay inspired every day. Gather images, quotes, and symbols that resonate with your business's objectives and desired outcomes. Place this board somewhere you will see it regularly, such as your workspace. This constant visual reminder helps reinforce your goals, maintain your motivation, and attract the opportunities and resources necessary to realize your vision.

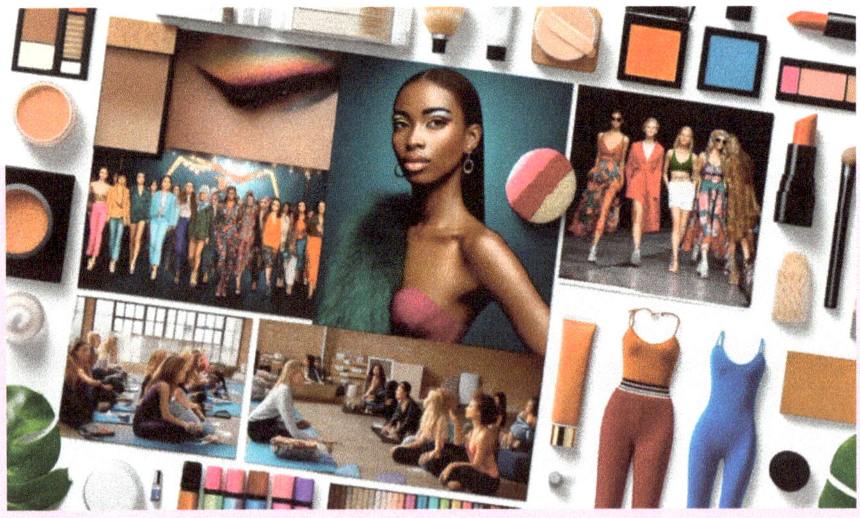

What are the top 4 things you want to accomplish in this industry?

☐ ______________________

☐ ______________________

☐ ______________________

☐ ______________________

chapter
07

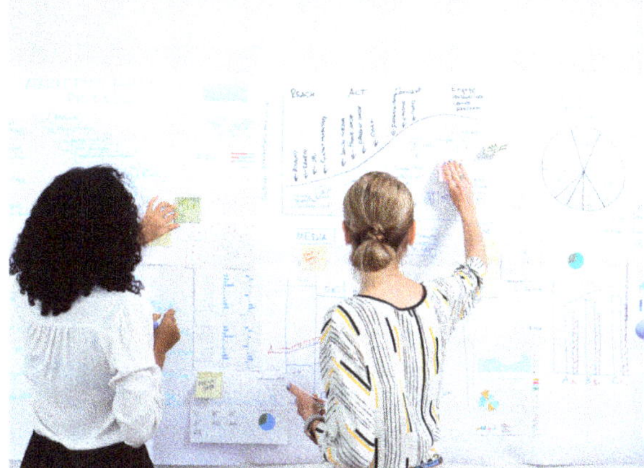

Establishing Your Brand in the Makeup Industry

In the makeup industry, who you know can be as important as what you know. This chapter focuses on how to effectively network and build relationships that can lead to career opportunities, collaborations, and growth.

Understanding Branding

Branding is more than just a logo or a color scheme; it's the entire identity of your business. It encompasses how you present yourself, your style of work, the values you communicate, and how clients perceive you.

Key Elements of Branding:

- **Unique Selling Proposition (USP)**: What makes you different from other makeup artists? It could be your specialization in a particular style, your approach to natural beauty, or your commitment to using eco-friendly products.

- **Visual Identity**: This includes your logo, color palette, and the overall aesthetic of your promotional materials.

- **Brand Voice:** The tone and language used in your communications, whether friendly and casual or sophisticated and professional.

Crafting Your Personal Brand

Define Your Audience

Understanding who your services are aimed at (e.g., brides, fashion models, everyday consumers) will guide how you market yourself and interact with potential clients.

Tell Your Story

Your background, experiences, and journey into makeup artistry can form a compelling narrative that resonates with your audience.

Consistency is Key

Ensure your visual identity and brand voice are consistent across all platforms, from your website to social media to physical marketing materials.

Effective Marketing Strategies

Marketing is crucial for attracting new clients and maintaining visibility in a saturated market.

Digital Marketing

- **Website**: Your website should be visually appealing, easy to navigate, and include a portfolio, your services, and contact information.

- **Social Media**: Platforms like Instagram and Facebook are powerful tools for showcasing your work, engaging with followers, and running targeted ads.

- **Email Marketing**: Build a mailing list and keep your subscribers engaged with updates, tips, promotions, and more.

- **Blogging**: Share makeup tips, product reviews, and industry insights to establish authority and drive traffic to your website.

- **Video Tutorials**: Posting tutorials on YouTube or Instagram can attract a following and showcase your expertise.

Networking and Partnerships

- Collaborations: Partner with other local businesses or influencers to expand your reach.
- Events: Participate in or sponsor beauty events and workshops to increase brand visibility and networking opportunities.

Leveraging Client Testimonials and Reviews

Positive feedback from clients builds trust and credibility.

- **Ask for Reviews**: Encourage satisfied clients to leave reviews on your website or social media pages.
- **Showcase Testimonials**: Feature testimonials prominently on your marketing materials and website.

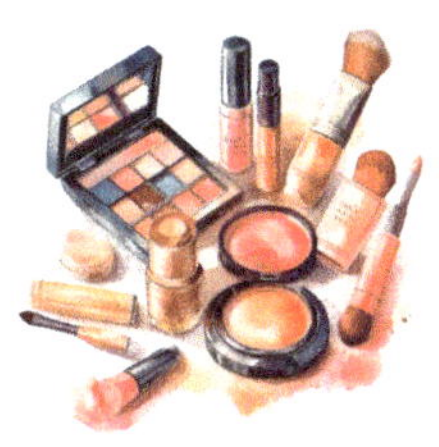

Overcoming Marketing Challenges

Staying Updated with Trends

The digital landscape is constantly evolving, requiring you to stay informed about the latest marketing trends and tools.

Budget Management

Effective marketing doesn't have to be expensive. Prioritize strategies that offer the best ROI, and use free or low-cost tools whenever possible.

Measuring Success

To understand the effectiveness of your marketing efforts, track metrics such as website traffic, social media engagement, and client inquiries.

Positive feedback from clients builds trust and credibility.

- Analytics Software: Use tools like Google Analytics for your website and native analytics on social media platforms.

- Feedback: Regularly solicit feedback from clients to learn what's working and what isn't.

Conclusion

Marketing and branding are ongoing processes that evolve with your business. By establishing a strong brand and implementing strategic marketing efforts, you can build a loyal client base and stand out in the competitive field of makeup artistry. Remember, the key to effective marketing is understanding your audience, communicating your unique strengths, and consistently delivering value.

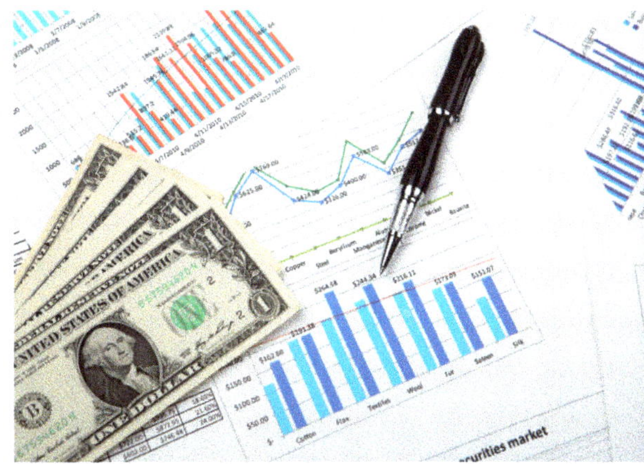

Navigating the Business Side of Makeup Artistry

In addition to your creative skills, effective financial management is crucial for the sustainability and growth of your makeup artistry business. This chapter provides insights into managing your finances, setting your pricing strategy, and ensuring profitability.

Understanding Basic Financial Management

The ability to manage your finances effectively is fundamental to running a successful business. It involves budgeting, tracking expenses, and making informed financial decisions.

Key Financial Concepts:

- **Budgeting**: Plan how to allocate your finances to cover various costs like supplies, marketing, and rent.

- **Expense Tracking**: Keep meticulous records of all business expenses to understand your financial flow and for tax purposes

- **Profit Analysis:** Regularly assess your profitability to adjust strategies and ensure business growth

Setting Up Your Financial Systems

Setting up the right systems from the start can save you time and help avoid financial issues down the road.

Tools and Resources:

- **Accounting Software**: Use software like QuickBooks or FreshBooks to simplify accounting processes and keep accurate records.

- **Financial Advisor**: Consider consulting with a financial advisor who understands small businesses to help set up your financial strategy.

- **Bank Accounts**: Open a separate bank account for your business to keep personal and business finances distinct.

Pricing Your Services

Determining how much to charge for your services is one of the most critical decisions you will make.

Factors Influencing Pricing:

- **Market Research**: Understand what competitors in your area charge for similar services.

- **Skill Level and Experience**: More experience or specialized skills generally justify higher rates.

- **Costs**: Include all costs (products, travel, time) in your pricing to ensure profitability.

Pricing Strategies:

- Hourly vs. Flat Rates: Decide whether you'll charge by the hour or by the project. Each has its advantages depending on the type of service you offer.
- Tiered Pricing: Offer different service levels to cater to a range of budgets.
- Packages: Create packages for events like weddings or photo shoots that offer multiple services at a bundled rate.

Managing Cash Flow

Effective cash flow management ensures you have enough money to cover business operations and avoid financial stress.

Tips for Managing Cash Flow:

- **Invoice Promptly**: Send invoices as soon as work is completed to ensure timely payments.

- **Deposit System:** Require deposits for bookings to secure the client's commitment and improve cash flow.

- **Emergency Fund**: Build an emergency fund to cover unexpected expenses or slow business periods.

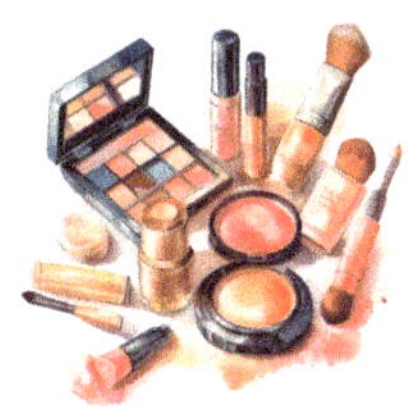

Tax Planning and Legal Considerations

Understanding your tax obligations and legal requirements is crucial to avoid penalties and ensure compliance.

Key Considerations:

- **Self-Employment Taxes**: Learn about your tax responsibilities as a self-employed individual, including estimated tax payments.

- **Business Licenses:** Ensure you have all necessary licenses to operate legally in your area.

- **Contracts:** Use contracts for client engagements to protect your interests and clarify expectations.

Investment and Growth

Investing back into your business is essential for growth and development.

Investment Areas:

- **Training and Education**: Continuously upgrade your skills and knowledge.

- **Quality Tools and Products**: Invest in high-quality makeup and tools to enhance your service offering.

- **Marketing**: Allocate budget for marketing to attract new clients and build your brand.

TAX-DEDUCTIBLE

Here's a comprehensive list of common small business expenses that you can typically claim on your taxes each year. Always consult with a tax professional to ensure compliance with current tax laws and regulations.

Office and Workspace Expenses

1. Rent or Lease Payments: Office space, studio, or storefront.
2. Utilities: Electricity, water, gas, internet, and phone bills.
3. Home Office Deduction: A portion of your home expenses if you use part of your home for business.
4. Office Supplies: Paper, pens, staplers, and other general office supplies.
5. Office Equipment: Computers, printers, phones, and other office machinery.

Business Operations

6. Professional Services: Accounting, legal, and consulting fees.
7. Insurance: Business insurance, including liability, property, and health insurance for employees.
8. Bank Fees and Interest: Fees for business bank accounts and credit card interest.

Marketing and Advertising

9. Advertising: Online ads, print ads, radio, and TV advertising.
10. Marketing Materials: Business cards, flyers, brochures.
11. Website and Hosting: Domain registration, hosting fees, and website maintenance.

Travel and Transportation

12. Business Travel: Airfare, hotel, meals, and transportation for business trips.
13. Vehicle Expenses: Mileage, gas, maintenance, and insurance for business vehicles.

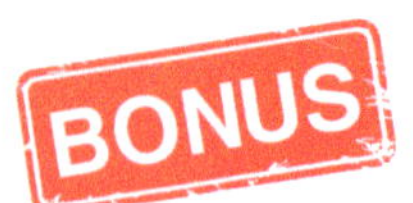

Employee and Contractor Expenses

1. Wages and Salaries: Payments to employees.
2. Contract Labor: Payments to independent contractors and freelancers.
3. Employee Benefits: Health insurance, retirement plans, and other benefits.

Meals and Entertainment

4. Business Meals: Meals with clients or potential business partners.
5. Entertainment: Limited deduction for entertainment expenses related to business.

Education and Training

6. Training Courses: Workshops, seminars, and courses related to your business.
7. Educational Materials: Books, subscriptions, and online courses.

Supplies and Inventory

8. Raw Materials: Items used to produce your products.
9. Finished Goods: Inventory for resale.

Licenses and Fees

10. Business Licenses: Licenses and permits required to operate your business.
11. Membership Dues: Professional associations and organizations related to your industry.

Depreciation

12. Depreciation: Deduction for the cost of business assets over time, such as equipment and vehicles.

Miscellaneous

13. Software and Subscriptions: Business-related software, cloud services, and subscriptions.
14. Postage and Shipping: Costs for mailing and shipping products or documents.

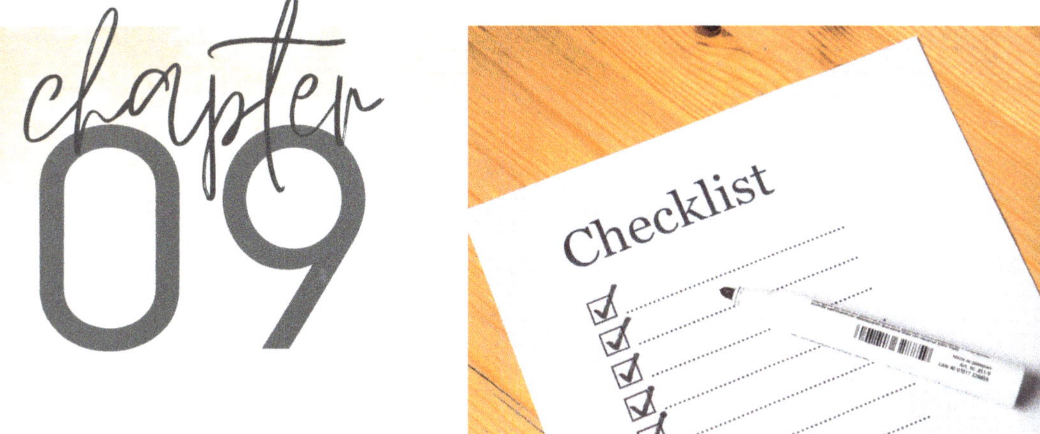

Laying the Foundation for Your Makeup Artistry Business

Starting a makeup artistry business requires careful planning and execution. This chapter provides a detailed checklist to help you establish and launch your business successfully.

Step 1: Develop a Business Plan

A well-thought-out business plan is crucial. It should outline your business goals, target market, services, pricing structure, marketing strategy, and financial projections.

Key Components:

- **Executive Summary**: A brief overview of your business and its objectives.

- **Market Analysis**: Insight into the makeup industry, your target audience, and competitors.

- **Services and Pricing**: Detailed descriptions of your services and pricing rationale.

- **Marketing and Sales Strategy**: How you plan to attract and retain clients.

- **Financial Plan**: Budgets, expected revenue, and financial goals.

Step 2: Choose a Business Structure

Decide on a legal structure for your business, such as sole proprietorship, partnership, LLC, or corporation. Each has different implications for liability, taxes, and ongoing requirements.

Considerations:

- **Legal Protection**: Some structures offer more personal liability protection than others.

- **Tax Implications**: Understand how each structure affects your taxes.

- **Ease of Setup**: Some structures are simpler and cheaper to set up than others.

Step 3: Register Your Business

Register your business with the appropriate local, state, and federal agencies. This includes obtaining any necessary licenses or permits.

Key Steps:

- **Business Name Registration**: Ensure your business name is available and register it.

- **EIN**: Obtain an Employer Identification Number from the IRS for tax purposes.

- **Permits and Licenses**: Check local regulations for any required permits or licenses.

Step 4: Set Up Your Financial Systems

Set up your accounting and financial management systems. This will help you keep track of income, expenses, and profitability.

Tools:

- Accounting Software: Choose software that fits your budget and business size.

- Business Bank Account: Open a bank account exclusively for business transactions.

- Budgeting: Create a budget to monitor and control financial activities.

Step 5: Acquire Equipment and Supplies

Purchase the necessary tools and products needed to provide your services. Quality and reliability are key when selecting your supplies.

Essentials:

- Professional Makeup Kit: High-quality products that cater to a variety of skin tones and types.

- Tools and Accessories: Brushes, sponges, and other application tools.

- Sanitation Supplies: Products to keep your tools clean and your practice sanitary.

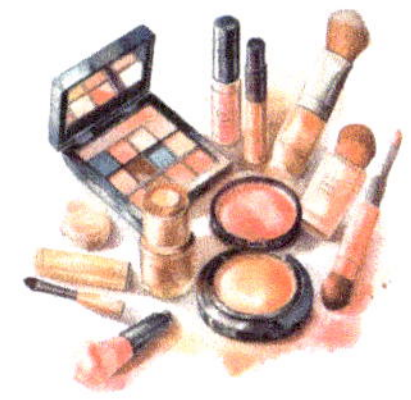

Step 6: Create Your Branding and Marketing Materials

Develop your branding, including a logo, business cards, and a website. Start creating content for your digital marketing campaigns.

Brand Identity:

- **Logo**: Create a logo that represents your brand's ethos.

- **Website**: Develop a professional website that showcases your portfolio and offers booking options.

- **Social Media**: Set up professional social media accounts to reach potential clients.

Step 7: Launch Marketing and Networking Efforts

Begin marketing your services through various channels. Attend networking events to connect with potential clients and other industry professionals.

Strategies:

- **Social Media Marketing:** Regular posts, ads, and engagement with followers.

- **Networking**: Join industry groups, attend local business events, and participate in community activities.

- **Referral Programs**: Offer incentives for clients who refer new customers.

Step 8: Start Taking Clients

Begin accepting clients. Focus on delivering excellent service to build a strong reputation and encourage repeat business and referrals.

Customer Service:

- **Quality of Work**: Ensure each client is satisfied with their makeup.

- **Professionalism**: Be punctual, organized, and courteous.

- **Follow-up**: Request feedback and thank clients for their business.

Step 9: Review and Adapt

Regularly review your business performance against your goals. Be prepared to adapt your strategy to meet market demands and grow your business.

Continuous Improvement:

- **Feedback:** Actively seek client feedback to improve your services.

- **Market Trends**: Stay updated on industry trends and adjust your offerings accordingly.

- **Financial Review**: Regularly review your financial status and adjust your budget and prices as necessary.

Conclusion

Launching your makeup artistry business involves multiple steps, from planning and registration to marketing and client management. By following this comprehensive checklist, you can establish a solid foundation for your business and position yourself for success in the competitive beauty industry.

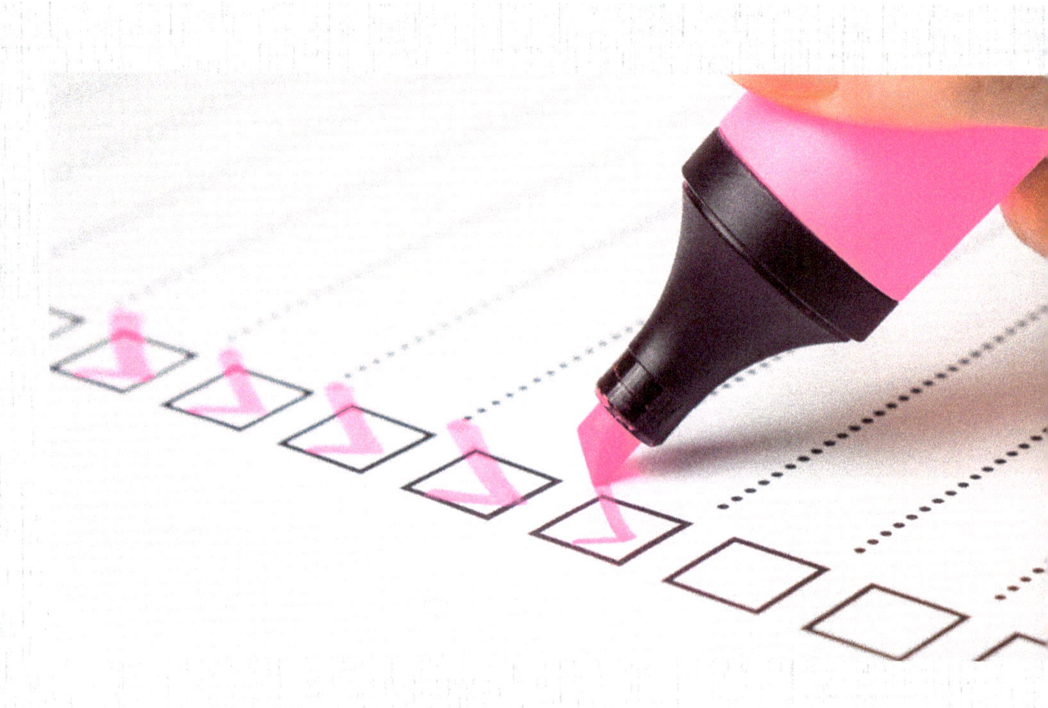

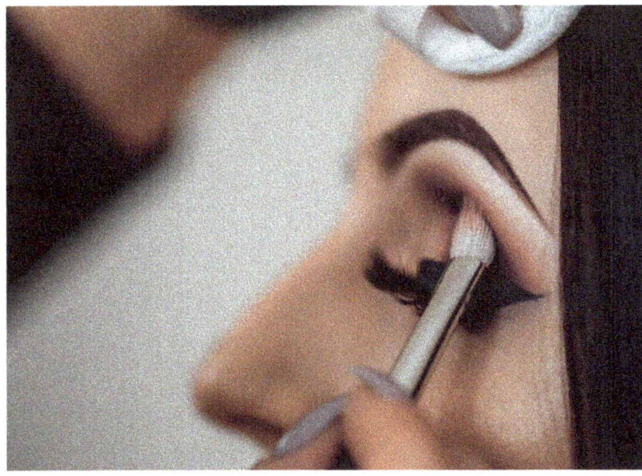

Reflecting on Your Journey and Looking Forward

Congratulations on reaching the final chapter of this comprehensive guide to becoming a successful makeup artist of color. This journey—from mastering the art of makeup to navigating the business world—is one of creativity, resilience, and continuous learning. As you move forward, keep in mind that your growth as a professional will be a dynamic process, shaped by both challenges and achievements.

Key Takeaways

Embrace Your Unique Identity

Your background and experiences are invaluable assets that add depth and perspective to your work. Celebrate and leverage your identity to differentiate yourself in the market and inspire your artistry.

Continuous Learning and Adaptation

The beauty industry is ever-evolving, with new trends, techniques, and products emerging regularly. Stay informed and adaptable, continuously refining your skills and expanding your knowledge to remain relevant and competitive.

Building Strong Relationships

The connections you make can open doors to new opportunities and provide support in your professional journey. Invest time in nurturing these relationships, and don't underestimate the power of a strong network.

Marketing and Branding Are Crucial

Your ability to market yourself and maintain a cohesive brand will greatly influence your success. Use the tools and strategies discussed to present a professional image and attract your target clientele.

Financial Discipline

Proper financial management is critical for the sustainability of your business. Keep diligent records, understand your expenses, and make informed decisions to ensure your business remains profitable and grows.

Future Growth and Opportunities

As you establish yourself in the industry, consider ways to expand your business and services. This might include:

- **Diversifying Services**: Offering classes, selling products, or specializing in niche areas like bridal or theatrical makeup.

- **Collaborating**: Working on projects with other artists or industries can provide new challenges and exposure.

- **Mentorship:** As you gain experience, consider mentoring new artists. This not only helps others but also enhances your reputation and expertise.

Staying Inspired

Your passion for makeup artistry was the spark that started this journey. Keep that passion alive by seeking inspiration in everything you do, whether through travel, art, fashion, or nature. Inspiration is the fuel that will keep your creative fires burning.

Giving Back

Consider using your skills and platform to contribute to your community and causes you care about. Whether it's offering free workshops for aspiring artists or supporting charitable events, giving back can be incredibly rewarding.

Final Thoughts

The path to becoming a successful makeup artist is as diverse as the individuals who embark on it. Your journey will be unique, filled with its own set of challenges and triumphs. Remember that every experience is an opportunity to learn, grow, and refine your craft.

Thank you for allowing this guide to be a part of your journey into the world of makeup artistry. Here's to your success, creativity, and the bright future that awaits you in the beauty industry!

Best of luck in your exciting and creative career!

MAKEUP LINE

Starting your own makeup line involves selecting the right vendors to ensure quality products and reliable service. Here are five vendors you might consider for sourcing ingredients, packaging, and manufacturing:

1. **Grafton Private Label Cosmetics** - Specializes in private label cosmetics, offering a wide range of makeup products that you can customize with your branding. They provide full-service options from product development to final packaging.

2. **Alibaba** - A global marketplace where you can connect with manufacturers for bulk ingredients and packaging materials. It's ideal for finding cost-effective solutions, though it requires careful selection and vetting of suppliers to ensure quality.

3. **Cosmetic Solutions** - This vendor offers turnkey solutions for beauty brands, including product formulation, manufacturing, and packaging. They are known for their innovation and high-quality products across various beauty categories.

4. **Beauty Manufacturing Solutions Corp (BMSC)** - Based in the USA, BMSC provides comprehensive services from product development to manufacturing and filling. They cater to both startups and established brands looking to expand their product lines.

5. **McKernan Packaging Clearing House** - Excellent for sourcing wholesale and surplus packaging components, such as bottles, jars, and caps. This can be a cost-effective option for startups needing quality packaging at lower volumes.

Each of these vendors offers unique strengths, so it's important to assess your specific needs regarding product formulation, budget, and quantity before making a decision.